ANGRY OCTOPUS

A Relaxation Story

BY LORI LITE

ILLUSTRATED BY
MAX STASUYK

Congratulations!

You are going to read a story called *Angry Octopus*. Follow the octopus along as he learns to calm down while he relaxes his mind and body. Notice how he learns to be the boss of his own feelings, body, and anger.

Note to Parent: Relaxation breathing works best when the belly rises with the breath coming in and the belly falls on the exhale. Do not overemphasize proper breathing. Bringing awareness to anger and breathing is already a big step. Enjoy!

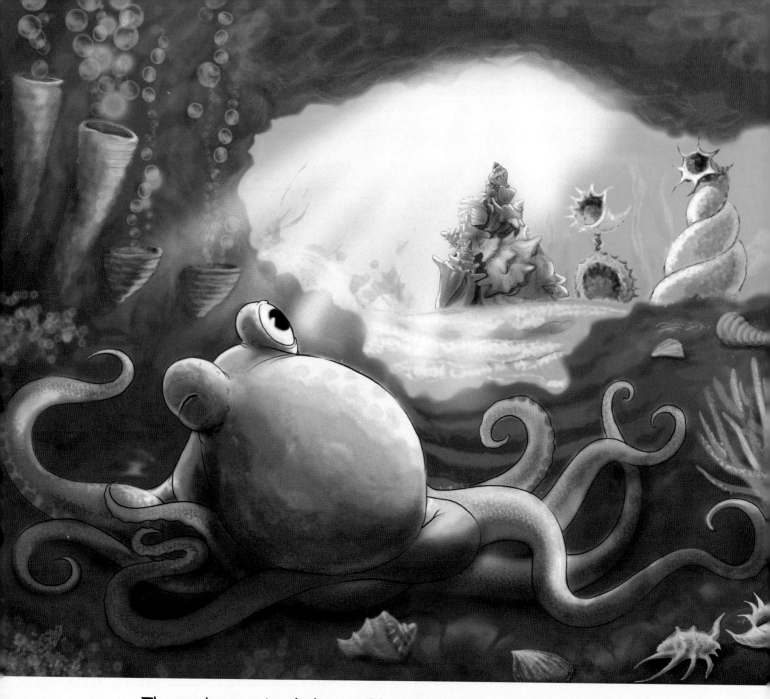

The sun's morning light trickled down through the water to the entrance of a cave. An octopus sleeping inside the cave could feel the life energy of the sun touch his face.

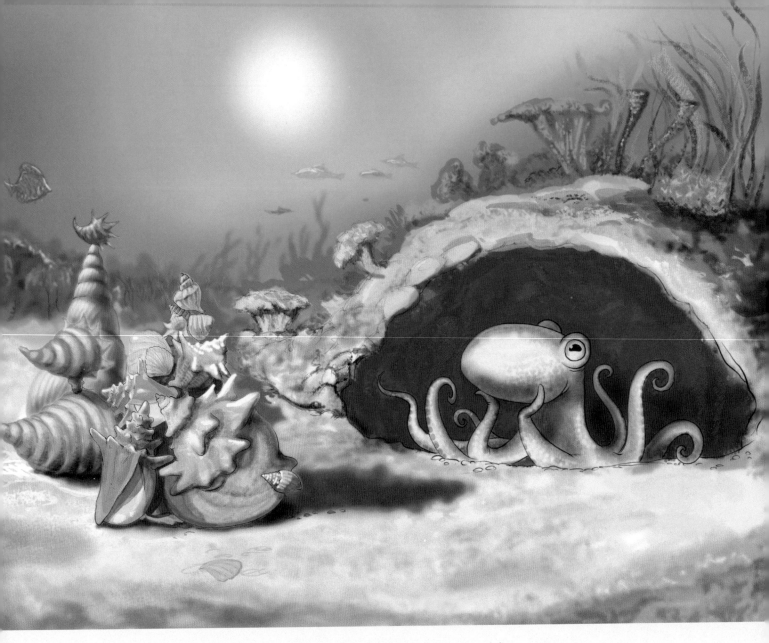

He took a deep breath and opened his eyes.
He stretched his body and ventured outside of his home. Just in front
of his cave was a seashell rock garden that he had created. Each morning
he would begin his day by eating breakfast in his special garden as he
watched the ocean come alive in the morning sun.

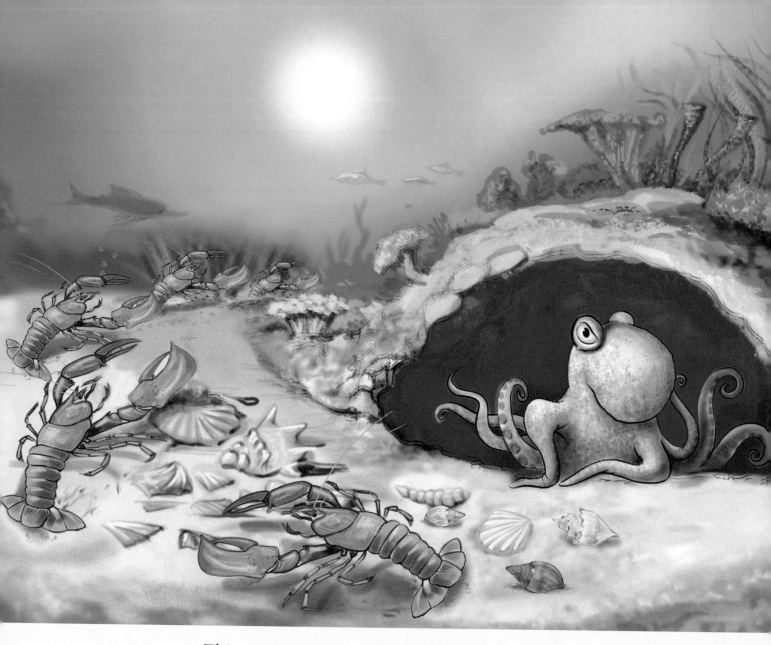

This morning his garden looked different.
During the night, lobsters traveling across the ocean floor had
bumped into his seashells and rocks. Everything was knocked over and
out of order. The octopus was not happy. In fact, he was very angry.

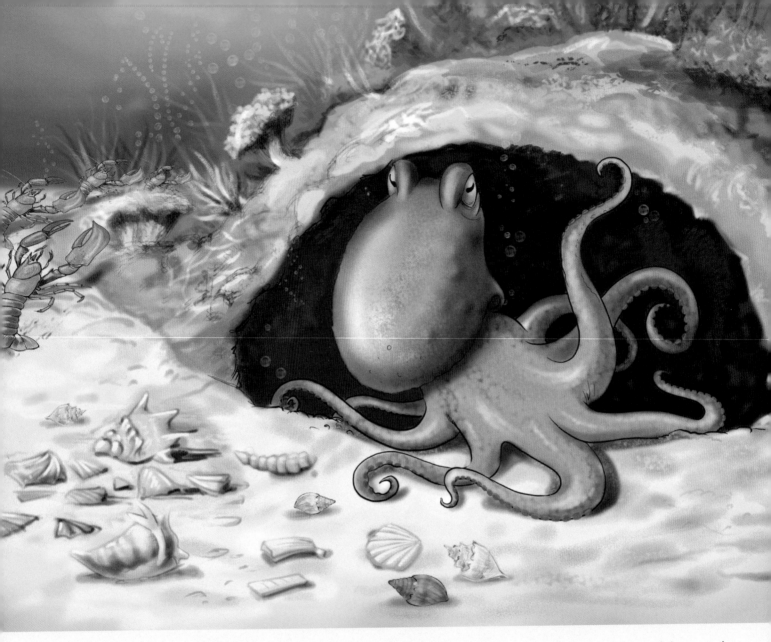

The more he looked at the mess the worse he felt. He got madder and madder and he felt his body get tighter and tighter. His muscles were tense and his stomach was rumbling like a volcano. He looked around at his ruined garden and his face started to turn red with anger. He knew what was happening to him but he did not know how to stop it. He was so angry that he thought he might explode... and, he did.

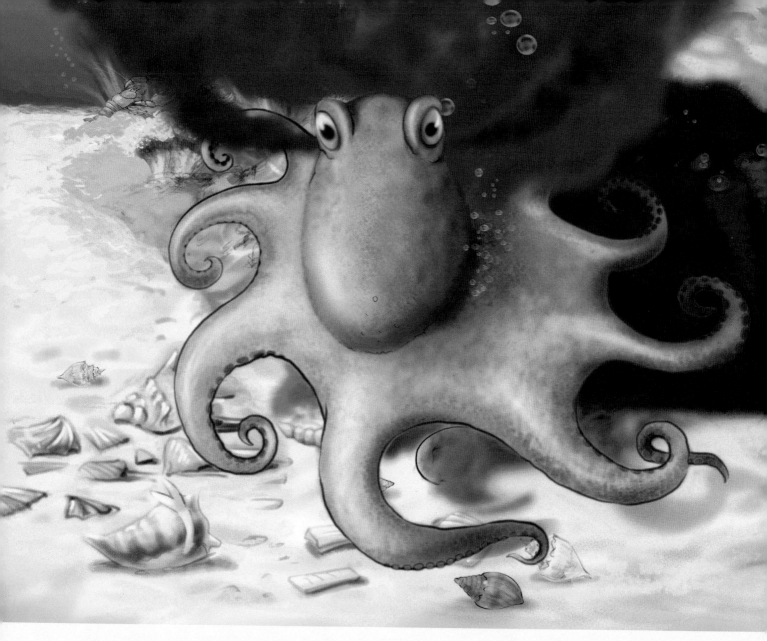

The angry octopus lost his temper, and as he screamed and yelled he
released a purplish-black cloud of ink into the water around him.
He felt frustrated and out of control. He didn't feel like he was the
boss of his own body or feelings, and now he couldn't see
through the dark ink cloud surrounding him.

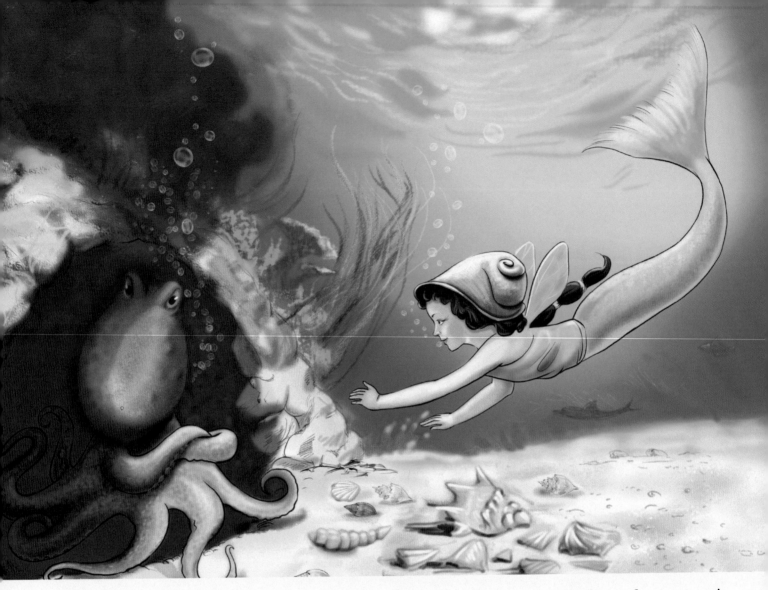

A sea child swimming by the cave saw the cloud of anger and confusion and stopped to speak to the octopus. "Why are you so angry? Why are you sitting in a dark cloud on such a beautiful day?" The octopus answered that he didn't know why he always did this when he got angry, but he did know that it didn't feel good to lose his temper and it always made his problem get worse.

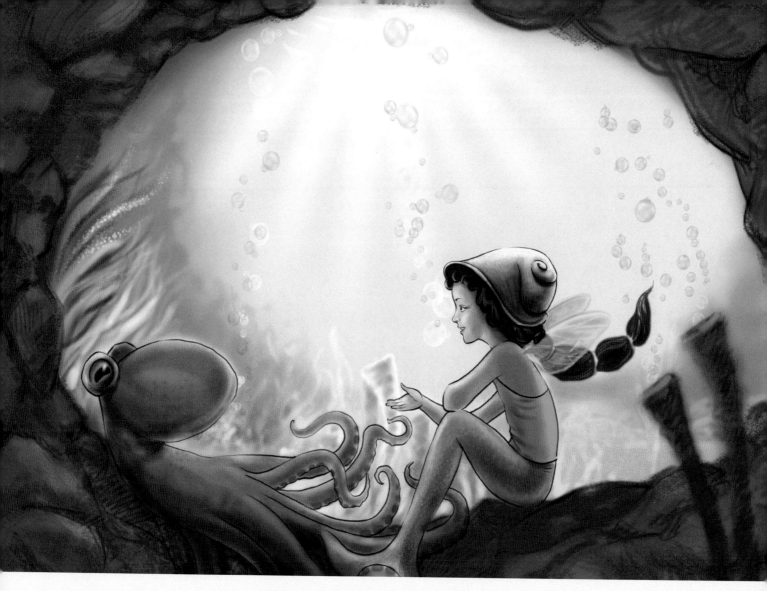

The sea child giggled and said,
"I will show you how to be the boss of your body and your anger. I will show
you how to calm down, let go of your anger, and see things more clearly."
"Lie down on your back and wiggle yourself into a comfortable position. Feel the sand
moving slowly around your body as you snuggle in. Now close your eyes and take a
deep breath. Breathe in through your nose and let the air out of your mouth..."
ahhh

"Now tighten your toes and feet. Squeeze them as tight as you can. Squeeze them into a tight ball."
Hold, hold, hold…

ahhh...
"Now let the air out of your mouth...
and let your toes and feet relax."
Surprisingly enough, the octopus felt
his toes and feet relax.

AAAHHHH!

The sea child continued,
"Tighten your legs tight as you can.
Squeeze them as tight as you can."
Hold, hold, hold...

ahhh...
"Now let the air out of your mouth... and let your legs stretch out gently as you let the angry, tight feelings start to slip away." The octopus felt his legs stretch out on the cool sand as he let the angry feelings leave his body.

AAAHHHH!

The sea child continued,
"Tighten your hips, stomach and back.
Squeeze them as tight as you can."
Hold, hold, hold...

ahhh...
"Now let the air out of your mouth...and let your back,
stomach and hips melt into the sand beneath you."
The octopus felt his body melting into the soft sand beneath him.
The rumbling in his stomach became quiet and was now replaced with
calm air as he felt his breath move in and out, in and out, in and out.

AAAHHHH!

The sea child continued,
"Tighten the muscles in your chest, your neck and shoulders.
Squeeze them as tight as you can."
Hold, hold, hold...

ahhh...
"Now let the air out of your mouth... and feel all that tension in your chest, neck and shoulders drift away." The octopus felt the tension leave his chest, neck and shoulders, and drift away.

AAAHHHH!

The sea child continued,
"Tighten your arms, hands and fingers. Squeeze them
as tight as you can. Squeeze them into a tight ball."
Hold, hold, hold...

ahhh...
"Now let the air out of your mouth... and let
your arms, hands and fingers unfold."
The octopus felt his hands open and the last
of his anger float away.

AAAHHHHH!

The sea child continued, "Tighten your jaw, your lips and your nose.
Crunch up your whole face. Squeeze them as tight as you can."
Hold, hold, hold...

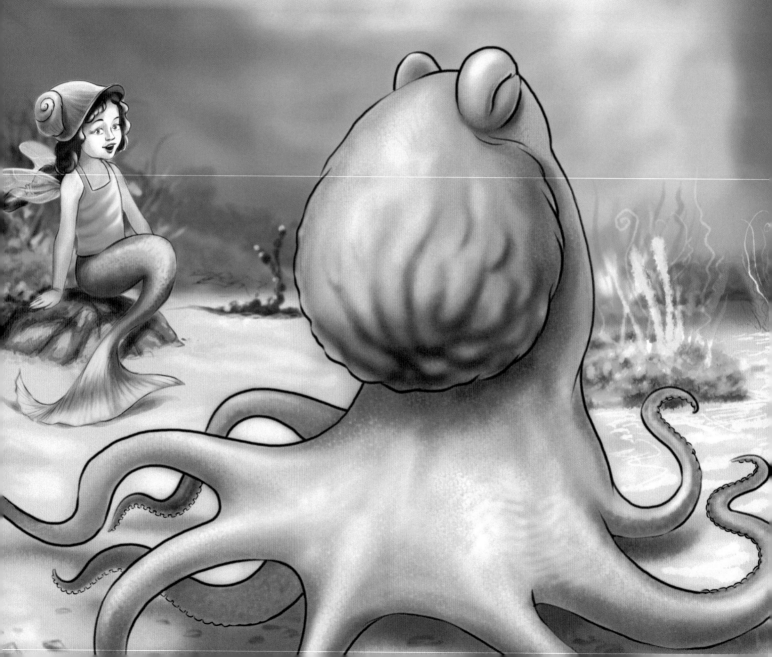

ahhh...

"Now let the air out of your mouth...and let your face and skin soften."
The octopus felt his skin soften. The octopus enjoyed how relaxed he
felt. He focused on how his breath was moving in and out, in and out,
in and out, filling his belly with warm, happy air.
He felt relaxed and peaceful.

AAAHHHH!

The sea child continued, "Tighten and wrinkle the skin on your forehead and the thoughts in your head. Squeeze them as tight as you can."

Hold, hold, hold...

ahhh...

"Now let the air out of your mouth...
and let your forehead and mind become
smooth and clear and still."

AAAHHHH!

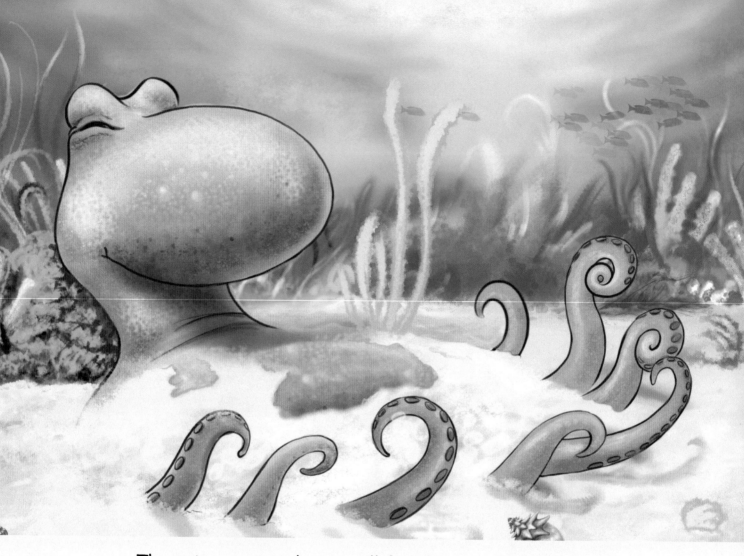

The octopus stayed very still for the next few moments.
He realized that he was now the boss of his own body and
feelings. He felt his breath moving in and out, in and out,
in and out touching every cell of his body.
He felt good.

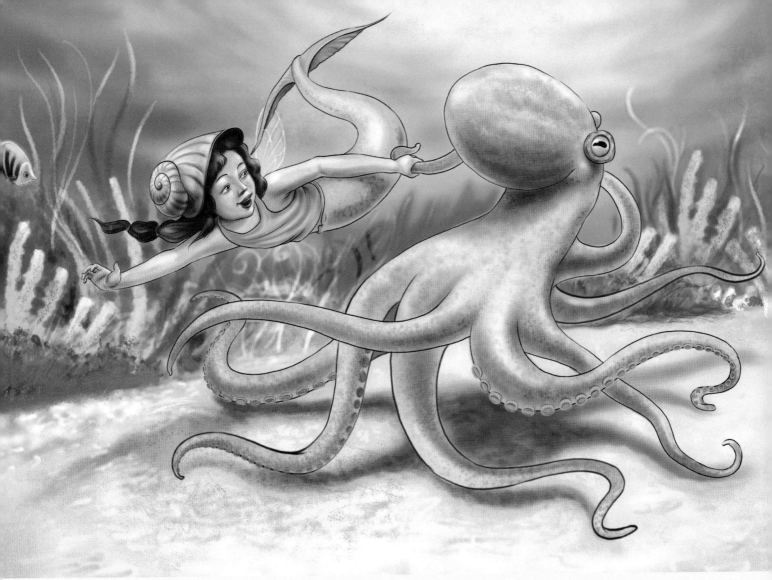

After a few moments, the octopus opened his eyes. His mood had shifted and the color of his body had returned to a warm shade of brown. He felt calm, balanced, and comfortable in his own skin. The dark cloud that had surrounded the octopus was gone. The ever moving ocean had replaced it with pure blue water. In this calm, still moment he realized that he could see things more clearly. He realized that he could solve his problem without being angry. With a little help he could fix his seashell rock garden.

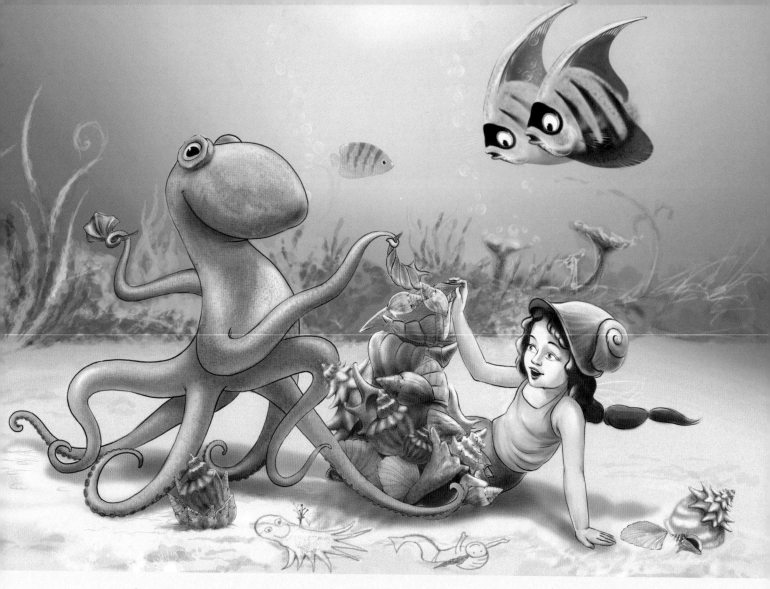

The octopus asked the seachild if she would help him. Together
they worked and laughed as they created a new seashell
rock garden that was more beautiful than anything he ever imagined.

Being the boss of his angry feelings helped the octopus to make a new friend.
Being calm helped him to see new possibilities.
It helped him to think clearly.

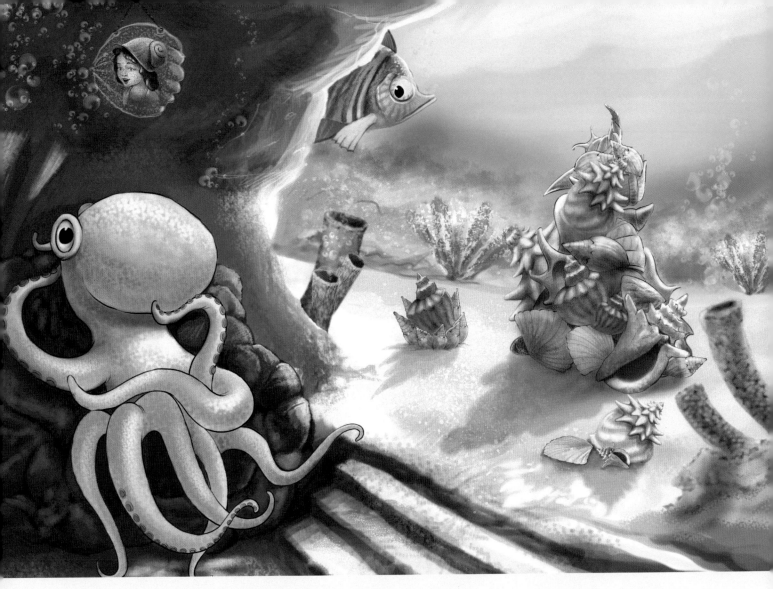

Now, whenever the octopus feels like he is going to explode with anger, he takes a deep breath...***ahhh.*** He tells himself that he is the boss of himself. He remembers that being calm helped him to fix his garden and make a new friend.

He smiles at how much better he feels, as he feels his
breath move in and out, in and out, in and out,
in and out, in and out, in and out...

Collect the Indigo Dreams Series and watch your whole family manage anxiety, stress and anger...

CD/Audio Books:

Indigo Dreams

Indigo Ocean Dreams

Indigo Teen Dreams

Indigo Dreams:
Garden of Wellness

Indigo Dreams:
Adult Relaxation

Indigo Dreams:
3 CD Set

Music CDs:

Indigo Dreams:
Kids Relaxation Music

Indigo Dreams:
Teen Relaxation Music

Indigo Dreams:
Rainforest Relaxation

Books:

The Goodnight Caterpillar

A Boy and a Turtle

Bubble Riding

Angry Octopus

Sea Otter Cove

Affirmation Weaver

A Boy and a Bear

The Affirmation Web

Resources:

Individual Lesson Plans

Stress Free Kids Curriculum

**Books, CDs and Lesson Plans are available at
www.StressFreeKids.com**

More Angry Octopus Fun

Angry Octopus Color Me Happy, Color Me Calm
A Self-Help Kid's Coloring Book for Overcoming Anxiety, Anger, Worry and Stress

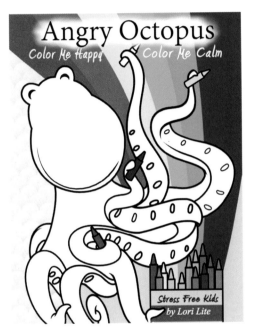

✓ Dozens of coloring pages designed for children.

✓ Underwater scenes, garden designs, Angry Octopus and friends, and a mandala.

✓ 38 self-soothing suggestions help relax, motivate, and introduce an anger or stress management technique in a playful manner.

This interactive coloring book is filled with simple strategies to self-soothe, manage anger, and improve emotional intelligence. Children are empowered to manage their BIG feelings.

Each mindful page motivates children to express themselves peacefully without having a tantrum, meltdown, or outburst.

Available on Amazon.com.
Take 15% off the price when purchasing from the StressFreeKids.com website by using Code AC59 at checkout.